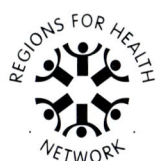 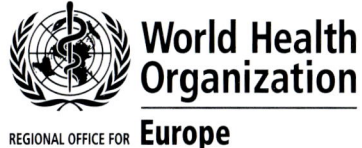

health equity
social sustainability
early-life conditions
education employment
participation
living habits
welfare

Tackling health inequities: from concepts to practice. The experience of Västra Götaland

Abstract

Despite remarkable health gains, inequities persist between and within countries in the WHO European Region and Sweden is no exception. Actions to effectively tackle health inequities need to be carried out at all levels of government. Regions have a key role to play in tackling health inequities in that they are close to their populations and have the power and skills to develop efficient public health policies that may contribute in reducing health disparities by changing the distribution of social determinants of health.

The report is about the process that the Region of Västra Götaland followed to mainstream the health equity dimension in its regional health plan and which resulted in the Action Plan for Health Equity in Region Västra Götaland. This publication is an account of the factors that made it possible, but it also presents a fair account of the obstacles encountered and the measures to overcome them. The report is a good illustration of how whole-of-government and whole-of-society approaches proposed by Health 2020 have been implemented in a real setting.

Keywords

INEQUALITIES
HEALTH POLICY
REGIONAL HEALTH PLANNING
SOCIAL DETERMINANTS OF HEALTH
SOCIOECONOMIC FACTORS

Address requests about publications of the WHO Regional Office for Europe to:
    Publications
    WHO Regional Office for Europe
    UN City, Marmorvej 51
    DK-2100 Copenhagen Ø, Denmark
Alternatively, complete an online request form for documentation, health information, or for permission to quote or translate, on the Regional Office web site (http://www.euro.who.int/pubrequest).

ISBN 978 92 890 5054 8
© World Health Organization 2014

All rights reserved. The Regional Office for Europe of the World Health Organization welcomes requests for permission to reproduce or translate its publications, in part or in full.

The designations employed and the presentation of the material in this publication do not imply the expression of any opinion whatsoever on the part of the World Health Organization concerning the legal status of any country, territory, city or area or of its authorities, or concerning the delimitation of its frontiers or boundaries. Dotted lines on maps represent approximate border lines for which there may not yet be full agreement.

The mention of specific companies or of certain manufacturers' products does not imply that they are endorsed or recommended by the World Health Organization in preference to others of a similar nature that are not mentioned. Errors and omissions excepted, the names of proprietary products are distinguished by initial capital letters.

All reasonable precautions have been taken by the World Health Organization to verify the information contained in this publication. However, the published material is being distributed without warranty of any kind, either express or implied. The responsibility for the interpretation and use of the material lies with the reader. In no event shall the World Health Organization be liable for damages arising from its use. The views expressed by authors, editors, or expert groups do not necessarily represent the decisions or the stated policy of the World Health Organization.

Edited by Nancy Gravesen
Book design by Marta Pasqualato
Printed in Italy by AREAGRAPHICA SNC DI TREVISAN GIANCARLO & FIGLI
Cover: © Göran Assner

CONTENTS

Foreword iv

Foreword vi

Acknowledgments vii

Executive summary 1

Section 1. Introduction 2

Section 2. Setting the scene 5
Regional organization in Sweden 5
The mandate 7

Section 3. Theoretical framework 10
The three domains 11
Kingdon's windows-of-opportunity theory 12
Actor-network theory and network formation theory 13

Section 4. Addressing health inequities in Västra Götaland 16
Motivation 16
Organizational structure 17
Phases 18
Action Plan 21
Influences on the Commission and its outcome 24

Section 5. Discussion 30

References 34

Foreword

It has been called the Swedish Paradox, the fact that, in spite of an advanced welfare society, health inequalities in Sweden have increased since the late 1970s. This is a phenomenon that Sweden shares with all European countries. The "Review of social determinants and the health divide in the WHO European Region" from 2013 showed that Europe has seen remarkable health gains, but inequities persist between and within countries. Regions have a key role in tackling health inequities in that they are close to their populations and have the power and skills to develop efficient public health policies that may contribute in reducing health disparities by changing the distribution of social determinants of health. However, we live in a complex society, and it is important to take advantage of scientific knowledge and practical experiences.

The global WHO Commission on Social Determinants of Health published a report "Closing the gap in a generation" that has been the inspiration for many nations, regions and cities all over the world to perform similar reviews albeit at a lower geographical level. Denmark, Norway and England (the United Kingdom) are but three examples at national level; in Sweden, the Malmö Commission, Region Västra Götaland, the Östgöta Commission and a joint collaboration coordinated by the Swedish Association of Local Authorities and Regions are examples of reviews or action plans developed at subnational level.

*Inspired by the WHO Commission, the Regional Executive Board in Västra Götaland assigned its Public Health Committee to produce an action plan to tackle the growing health inequalities within the region. It should be developed **together** with relevant stakeholders in Västra Götaland and aim at **concrete** actions that could be implemented within a short timeframe.*

*This report is about the process that led to the final action plan, now approved by the Regional Council, and thus an important document for public health in Västra Götaland. It is an account of the achievements but also of the mistakes we have experienced during the process. I think that the process we have been running is a good illustration of the WHO strategy Health 2020 **in practice**. Health 2020 has proved to be valuable and useful for us as health policy-makers, not only providing us with a theoretical framework to organize our work but also giving legitimacy to our arguments. By accounting for the lessons we have learnt and by sharing them with you, we wish to contribute to the capacity-building mentioned in Health 2020 as a priority area.*

This is, indeed, a good example of how regions might benefit from collaborating with WHO and, hopefully, how WHO might find it useful to collaborate with regions to strengthen and enrich the social movement against health inequities initially suggested by Sir Michael Marmot (Professor, Epidemiology and Public Health, University College, London, United Kingdom and Chair of the WHO Commission on Social Determinants of Health) and now taking shape. Therefore, I wish to express my sincere gratitude to the WHO Regional Office for Europe and its WHO European Office for Investment for Health and Development in Venice, Italy for their unfailing support in our endeavour to fight back the unfair inequalities in health that, to a growing extent, are limiting the capabilities of so many people to be healthy, thereby threatening a sustainable development for us all.

Jan Alexandersson
Chair, Public Health Committee
Region Västra Götaland
Sweden

Foreword

Health 2020 was adopted in September 2012 by the 53 Member States of the WHO European Region. Built on solid evidence, the policy framework for health and well-being represents a watershed in the European public health scene. It sets clear goals to improve populations' health and clearly identifies strategic areas of action. The unanimous endorsement of Health 2020 put the spotlight on the serious problem of health inequities. Health 2020 has contributed to place them at the top of the political agenda of European countries.

Many of the actions to tackle health inequities are taken at the subnational level of governance, especially in those countries with a high level of devolution. It is often at this level that initiatives are taken and scaled up to the national level.

Thanks to an incredible variety of socioeconomic contexts and political and institutional arrangements, the WHO European Region is a huge repository of processes, policies and interventions implemented to confront various health challenges. Health inequities are no exception. The body of knowledge in terms of measures to tackle them in the European Region is substantial.

With this publication, the WHO Regional Office for Europe focuses on the process of incorporating the equity dimension into regional health planning by describing the experience of the Swedish Region of Västra Götaland.

This publication offers a bird's eye view of the overall problem of health inequities and, equipped with a broader overview of the different stakeholders that come to play in various institutional arrangements, then it delves into specific topics. These include theoretical frameworks, possible organizational structures and systems to increase ownership and accountability of the involved stakeholders. These elements are complemented by a checklist, which helps readers understand where they stand on the pathway to ensure that reducing health inequities is part of their regional health planning process.

Translating theories on how to tackle health inequities and on how to foster proactive intersectoral collaboration into practice is the essence of this publication.

I am convinced that the process used by Region Västra Götaland and described in this publication will be inspirational to many regions and, as such, will substantially contribute to advance health, equity and well-being in Europe.

Erio Ziglio
WHO Focal Point, Regions for Health Network
Head, WHO European Office for Investment for Health and Development
WHO Regional Office for Europe

Acknowledgments

The WHO Regional Office for Europe thanks members of Region Västra Götaland and the Public Health Committee for their willingness to share their experience with other countries and regions. It also thanks all stakeholders mentioned in this publication for their contribution to the whole-of-government approach that led from a political commission to a comprehensive policy plan.

Thanks go to Gustaf Kastberg (Lund University and Municipality Research in western Sweden), who evaluated the process and has provided extensive information for this report; the WHO Regions for Health Network members: Chris Riley (Welsh Government, United Kingdom), Kai Michelsen (Maastricht University, the Netherlands) and Solvejg Wallyn, (Flemish Ministry of Welfare, Public Health and Family, Belgium) who provided critical expert review of the draft document; Mary Jo Monk (Government of Nova Scotia, Canada) for providing input on the Social Policy Framework for Nova Scotia; and Sara Barragan Montes (WHO Regional Office for Europe) for providing pictures for the report.

The report was written by Maria Berhe and Göran Henriksson (Public Health Secretariat in Region Västra Götaland) with Francesco Zambon (WHO Regional Office for Europe). Special thanks go to Region Västra Götaland for its continued support of the work of the WHO European Office for Investment for Health and Development of the WHO Regional Office for Europe, as well as to the WHO Regions for Health Network, for making this publication possible.

Executive summary

This publication, produced by Region Västra Götaland and the WHO Regional Office for Europe, adds to the growing number of reports on joint efforts to tackle health inequalities. Governance for equitable health requires the involvement of a broad spectrum of stakeholders as well as contextual flexibility for framing the problem. The joint venture to create an action plan for social sustainability and health equity in Västra Götaland, Sweden serves as an example of the pitfalls and the possibilities of collaborative processes.

The following key messages could be useful to other regions, countries and municipalities that are beginning their own joint ventures to tackle health inequalities.

Be aware of the so-called window of opportunity and identify the steps an organization can take to raise awareness in the organization at large, as well as in the eye of the public. For a fruitful joint effort, it is important to converge the problem, the policy and the political stream.

Build the venture on a clear political mandate from regional/national/local government and make sure to anchor the work along the way. An inclusive process (whole-of-government approach) might result in future questions such as: what are the decision forums for implementation? Are all levels of the delivery chains on board, who will prioritize actions and how will they be prioritized? All these questions need to be dealt with at the political level and preferably early on in the process.

For future implementation, it is also imperative to **gather relevant stakeholders and find a common language**. This is a necessary step that should occur prior to setting a common goal for the venture and understanding the roles and responsibilities for all stakeholders (whole-of-society approach).

For the process to be able to include these messages, **set a timeline that allows for consultation, negotiation, anchoring and decision-making**. That also leaves time, for example, to enrol hard-to-reach stakeholders and/or forge links to other strategic documents currently in force or in the planning process.

Section 1. Introduction

Even if the health of the population in Västra Götaland is generally good, there are still significant inequalities in health and in the distribution of social determinants. It is especially worrying that inequalities in health in some aspects have increased during the past three decades. One example is life expectancy at age 30 for women, which has been increasing from 52 years in 1986 to 54 years in 2010 (1). However, *the divide* between women with low educational attainment and those with high educational attainment has increased from 2 years in 1986 to 4.2 years in 2010. Another example is excess premature deaths. According to a recent study, there are 1600 premature deaths in Västra Götaland each year among the population aged 25–74 years (approximately 920 000) due to socioeconomic inequalities (2). Given the reputation that Sweden, as well as the other Nordic countries, has for doing well in terms of equity (this is indeed so in terms of absolute differences), the growing inequalities might seem paradoxical. Why does not a growing welfare and prosperity translate into reduced inequalities in health?

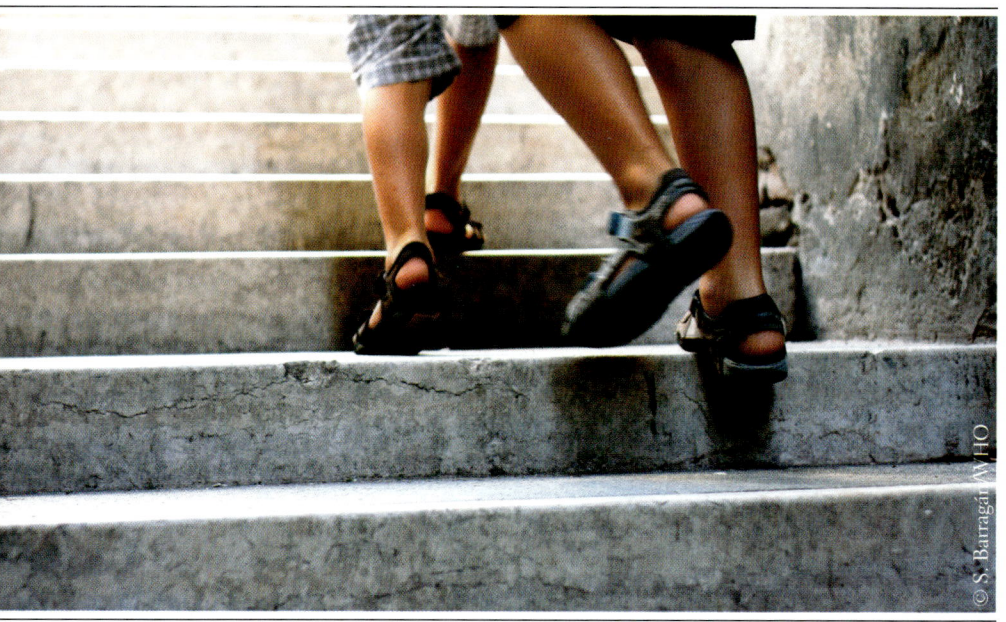

Health inequalities mirror the conditions under which people grow, live, work and age and, as stated in the final report of the WHO Commission on Social Determinants of Health, these conditions are, in turn, shaped by political, social and economic forces (3). As a consequence, tackling health inequalities requires joint action by multiple actors and stakeholders. It is necessary to look at the process of policy-making, how decisions are made that might influence the distribution of the social determinants of health and the response in terms of implementation and effects on the distribution of health in the population.

Following the launch of the final report from the WHO Commission on Social Determinants of Health in late 2008 (3), the Regional Council in Region Västra Götaland decided to start a joint venture to tackle inequalities in health in its Region. The challenge was to identify actions that should be efficient and concrete, and also to attract different stakeholders with different agendas and objectives to make a joint effort to tackle health inequalities within the region and, at the same time, have political commitment to the work.

This report aims to summarize the process, which evolved as a result from the Regional Council's decision. Section 2 presents a short background on how the process began, and Section 3 gives an account of the theoretical framework that served as a compass for the process. Section 4 describes the process and the *Action Plan for Health Equity in Region Västra Götaland (4)* and provides an analysis on success factors as well as pitfalls. The last section is a discussion in which certain important parts of the process are highlighted.

This report adds to the growing number of reports on joint efforts to tackle health inequalities, such as the Norwegian case (5) and *Malmö's path towards a sustainable future (6)* in Sweden. These reports might inspire others to launch similar local and regional processes. An underlying theme in these reports is governance – the idea that interdependence among societal actors requires joint action to make a difference – a core message in the WHO Health 2020 strategy (7). This report illustrates a regional effort to establish a network of stakeholders, based on previous reviews on health inequities.

Even if there can be no universal solution that works in all contexts, a strategy to reduce health inequalities must recognize the complexity in modern societies, which are increasingly interdependent in a globalized world and thus require new approaches to governance where key goals include political support for health equity as a societal good, the coherence of actions across sectors and stakeholders, and an improvement in the distribution of opportunities to be healthy, across the whole population *(8)*.

Section 2. Setting the scene

This publication presents the experiences from Region Västra Götaland's work with its commission to tackle health inequalities. To be of use for other regions and stakeholders, it is important to describe the Region and its functions and an overview is in Box 1.

Box 1. Quick facts

Region Västra Götaland (the organization) is:

- the result of merging three county councils and parts of the city of Göteborg in 1999;
- responsible for health care and medical treatment;
- responsible for growth and development matters;
- operates with costs of approximately 40 billion Swedish kronor; and
- employs approximately 50 000 people.

Region Västra Götaland (the territory) has:

- 1.5 million inhabitants;
- 49 municipalities;
- Göteborg as its largest city;
- the largest port in Scandinavia;
- the status of Sweden's leading region for industry and transportation; and
- 23% of the population with at least 3 years tertiary education, the same level as Sweden in general, which varies between 11% and 31% when looking at geographical differences.

Source: adapted and reproduced by permission from Region Västra Götaland (4,9).

REGIONAL ORGANIZATION IN SWEDEN

PUBLIC ADMINISTRATION

Sweden has three formal levels of public government: the state at national level, the municipalities at local level and the regions in between. Legislation is the main responsibility of the state, thus forming the framework of the welfare institutions. The municipalities are responsible to a large extent to deliver these core welfare institutions such as schools, child care, elderly care, etc. The municipality has a high level of autonomy versus the state and the region and may decide, within the legal framework provided by the Riksdag (Swedish Parliament), how to allocate the available resources. They also have the right to decide on taxes. The region, as a governmental structure between the state and the municipality, is responsible by law for the organization of health care but has also taken over some of the authorities from the state, such as regional infrastructure, transportation and creating opportunities for sustainable growth. The Regional Council also has the right to decide on taxes.

Internal organizational structures and mandates

The regional administrative organization is thus part of a fairly decentralized governmental structure in Sweden, sharing the responsibility to organize major parts of the welfare institutions with the municipalities.

The public health sector within the regional administration is divided into two parts, the Public Health Committee, and the Health and Medical Care Committees (HMCCs). Whereas the former is a political committee serving directly under the Regional Executive Board on strategic public health issues, the latter is a decentralized political entity responsible for organizing local health care and public health (from 2015 onwards there will be five such HMCCs). They are accountable to the Regional Council and a part of the purchaser–provider system (Fig. 1).

Since the health care sector in the region is organized under a purchaser-provider system, the operative public health organization is administered by the HMCCs, responsible for both health care and public health. Due to the autonomy of the municipalities, local public health plans are negotiated between the regional "purchasers" and each municipality.

Fig. 1. Political organization of Region Västra Götaland

```
                          ┌─────────────┐
                    ┌────→│  Regional   │
                    │     │   Council   │
                    │     └─────────────┘
┌─────────────┐     │     ┌─────────────┐
│  Health and │     │     │  Regional   │←─────────┐
│ medical care│           │Executive Board│         │
└─────────────┘           └─────────────┘   ┌───────────────────┐
                                 ↑ ↑        │ Regional development│
                                 │ │        │ (Purchaser and     │
                                 │ │        │ provider system    │
                                 │ │        │ within regional    │
                                 │ │        │ development – divided into│
                                 │ │        │ subareas)          │
                                 │ │        └───────────────────┘
┌─────────────┐         ┌─────────────┐          ┌─────────────┐
│  Health and │         │Public Health│          │  Regional   │
│ Medical Care│         │ Committee   │─────────→│ Development │
│  Committee  │←───────→│(Strategic advisory│    │  Committee  │
│(Purchaser and│        │ board within the public│└─────────────┘
│provider system within│ │ health area)│
│health and medical│    └─────────────┘
│care as well as public│        ↑↓
│    health) │          ┌─────────────┐          ┌─────────────┐
└─────────────┘         │ Human Rights│          │Cultural Affairs│
                        │  Committee  │─────────→│  Committee  │
                        └─────────────┘          └─────────────┘
```

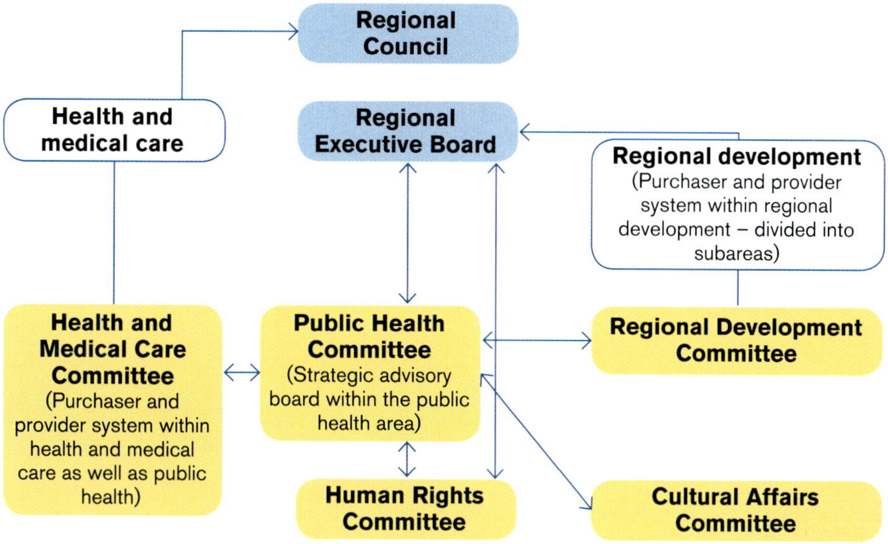

Source: adapted and reproduced by permission from Region Västra Götaland *(10,11)*.

The mandate

In light of the WHO Commission on Social Determinants of Health, as well as other events,[1] the Regional Council, in 2010, commissioned the Public Health Committee to coordinate work to produce a regional action plan to reduce health inequalities within the region. The Commission to create an Action Plan for Health Equity in Västra Götaland, hereafter referred to as the Commission, should base its work on the conclusions from the previous work of the WHO Commission.

A Political Steering Group, hereafter referred to as the Steering Group, was formed and agreed on a target and scope for the action plan:

> *to contain proposals of concrete initiatives/measures – locally, regionally and nationally – which are most likely to reduce health inequity in Västra Götaland. Each actor then decided in their own organization on which of the proposed initiatives/measures should be implemented, as well as when and how they should be implemented. (4)*

---

[1] A more comprehensive description of motivations that led to this process is in Section 4.

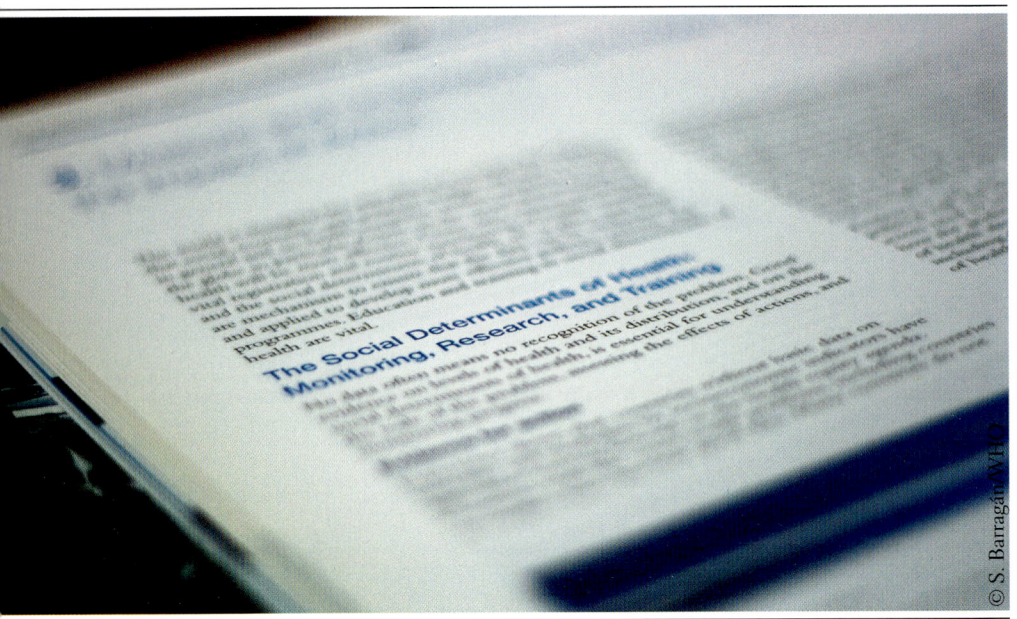

One might comment on the fact that a regional action plan contains proposals for local as well as national arenas, both autonomous levels. This way of emphasizing situations and initiatives that require collaboration across different levels of society is necessary in order to include the root causes as well as the different welfare systems that, to a great extent, affect the health status of citizens. As the Steering Group stated, the regional level can work from mandates provided by the Steering Group, but the national level needs to provide the Steering Group with better tools. This does not imply that Region Västra Götaland can decide on actions to be taken on any other level than its own.

Clearly this scope presumes a new approach to collaboration where different stakeholders, each with their own agenda and responsibilities for the health and welfare of the population, are supposed to coordinate their efforts to tackle health inequalities within their own scope for action. Such a collaborative network is an example of *governance* structure rather than *government* organization.

Kickbusch and Gleicher *(12)* refer to such a governing strategy to tackle health inequalities as "smart governance", characterized by governing:

- by collaboration
- through citizen engagement
- through a mix of regulation and persuasion
- through independent agencies and expert bodies
- through adaptive policies, resilient structures and foresight.

Section 3. Theoretical framework

This section presents some tools used to explain what decisions were made during the process, the different roads chosen and how the process led to the final Action Plan *(4)*. During the initial planning phase, the theories used were more of a methodological character, such as the Delphi process *(13)* used to identify and develop the *situations* that should be tackled and the corresponding actions that might impact on the *situations*. But this theoretical framework can, in retrospect, clarify what happened.

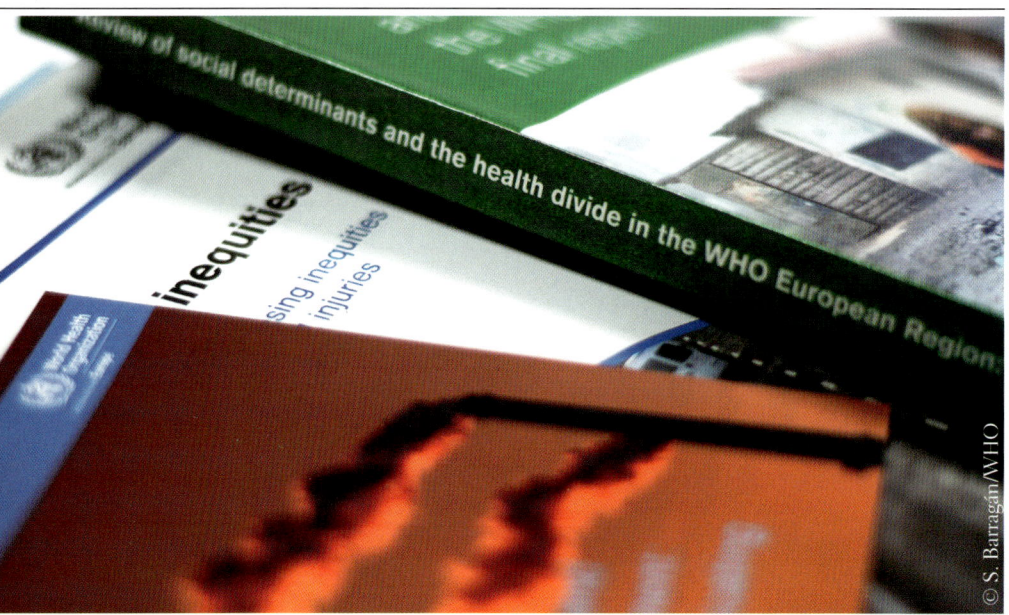

Several scholars have pointed to the complexity in transforming public health evidence into practice. Tackling inequalities in health is no exception. The structural transformation of society in general during the last decades has gone from a more uniform and sectored organization, where the municipalities and the state played a dominant decision-making role, towards a more complex situation with more decision-making levels where decisions made at one level might influence the effects from decisions made at other levels. Public administrations are no longer free to decide without considering other decision-making bodies and, at the same time, their decisions and the efficiency of the implementation of their decisions will depend on decisions made by other bodies. Failures to implement a certain strategy or actions are thus not necessarily due to what happens in one's own organization but could well be the result from strategies and decisions at other levels by other actors *(14)*.

This is a main reason as to why a common recommendation for work within the field of public health is to emphasize coordination and concerted action by many different stakeholders within the scientific, public, professional and civic societies *(8)*. To develop the Action Plan, it was necessary to organize and collaborate with a network of actors in the Region.[2] In the following section, the three domains that together form human service organizations are described to better understand the limitations and possibilities inherent in the collaborative network that evolved in the regional process. It is clear that a decision is not the result of a linear procedure but rather from a situation where a number of conditions coincide, by chance or deliberately. The process itself was evaluated using an actor-network theory to analyse the development process and to identify successes and mistakes. The core of this theory is also accounted for.

THE THREE DOMAINS

In their often cited paper, Kouzes and Mico suggest that human service organizations comprise three distinct domains – policy, managment and service – rather than an all-including hierarchy and a linear decision-making process *(15)*. Each of the three domains operates by different principles and rationales, measures of success, work mode and structures (Table 1). These conflicting principles are important explanatory factors to understand the difficulties that emerge when political decisions are to be implemented into action.

Table 1. The three domains of human service organizations

Domain	Principles	Success measures
Policy	Consent of the governed	Equity
Management	Hierarchical control and coordination	Cost efficiency and effectiveness
Service	Autonomy and self-regulation	Quality of service, good standards and practice

Source: information based on Kouzes & Mico *(15)*.

---

[2] An overview of the organizations involved is in Section 4.

These three domains do not include all stakeholders in the process but exemplify the difficulties one might face when having to create a platform for joint ventures due to different principles and measures of success. The basic principle of the policy domain is consent of the governed, as expressed in democratic and fair elections of representatives who vote, bargain and negotiate. The basic principle of the management domain is hierarchical control and coordination to use distributed resources in a cost-effective and efficient way. Its structure is bureaucratic and the administrators use linear techniques and tools to produce results. The service domain is characterized by its relative autonomy by professionals whose objectives are to achieve good quality and standards of practice to best benefit their clients. Their services are based on expertise and knowledge about mechanisms underlying the phenomena in focus, be they diseases or poverty or something else.

All three domains are crucial to implement a certain decision and, at the same time, often conflict. It therefore is important to consider how these domains will react when trying to implement an action plan to reduce health inequalities and not assume a priori that decisions are implemented in a linear process from politics to action.

Why is it often very difficult to develop and agree on a comprehensive and coordinated policy and even more difficult to implement it, in spite of an agreement that the objective is "is to create societal prerequisites for good health on equal terms for the entire population" *(16)*, as in the Swedish national public health policy goal? Part of the answer is that there are a number of different interpretations of what is meant by concepts like equity, health and social conditions and how these are turned into momentum in policy and political arenas: within the three (conflicting) domains.

KINGDON'S WINDOWS-OF-OPPORTUNITY THEORY

Everyone with a little experience with policy-making acknowledges that decisions seldom if ever come through the classical linear decision-making process, which starts with a mapping of possible solutions, their prioritization and proper implementation, and concludes with adequate evaluation for efficiency. Such a linear decision-making process is rather a Weberian "ideal type". In practice, decision-making is a lot more complex undertaking.

Kingdon has offered an explanation in his windows-of-opportunity theory (17). He suggests that decisions are about the timing and flow of three streams: the problem stream, the policy stream and the political stream. Each has its own dynamic and is largely independent, with actors within each of the streams that can meet and sometimes overlap. It is the occasions when the three strands converge and link a problem with a solution (policy) that is politically feasible, that the windows of opportunity open.

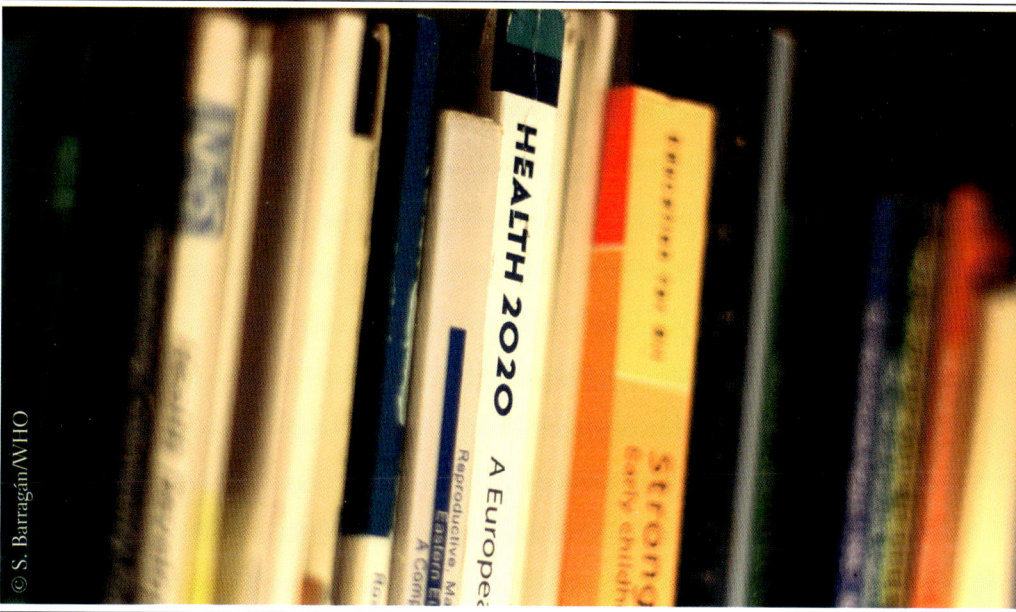

Such links often occur via policy entrepreneurs, people who "invest their resources in return for future policy they favour" (17). Examples include politicians, researchers, leaders in business or governments or significant persons in the public eye. The sector and role of policy entrepreneurs are to define problems and link them to political agendas by acting as so-called translators and facilitate collaboration between stakeholders, using formal and informal approaches.

ACTOR-NETWORK THEORY AND NETWORK FORMATION THEORY

When using actor-network theory to analyse processes, the focus lies on negotiations, creating relationships and the tools used. One conclusion from later research on strategies is that an action plan is but one point in a process that begins before the final version is presented and, hopefully, will continue a long time thereafter (18). It is often difficult to disentangle the different phases in a strategic process, and the development of the action plan is often a tool used in parallel with other activities that enhance the implementation of the action plan.

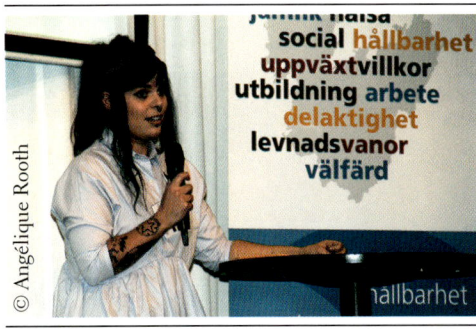

It has been suggested that an action plan expresses what has been labelled a visualization. Visualization is a description of reality, a map, which many actors regard as a true representation of reality (18). This is a valuable concept since it creates a distinct relationship between the negotiation process leading to the visualization and the effects that could be expected from the implementation of the visualization. If there is no agreement that the action plan describes reality in a realistic way, then it should not be expected to have an impact at a later stage.

The concept of visualization also makes the actors participating in the process visible and makes the factors that create the network of actors important.

According to the actor-network theory, actors within a network have their own interests and agendas and will try to pursue these. This means that collaboration requires the collaborators to think it is meaningful to collaborate because they will gain something, which they believe is valuable or useful. Thus, the formation of the network is crucial to make the action plan based on collaboration a significant document.

This formation of a network can, according to Callon (19), be captured by four concepts.

- *Problematizing* is about actors sharing a common definition of a problem and who think it is useful to collaborate to solve the problem. This is not only a central part in forming and establishing a network but also important later in the process when new actors have been identified.

- *Interessement* is about how actors are recruited to the network and what makes them decide to participate. It could be about pointing to the advantages and wins with participating, but it could also be about using power or force to ensure participation.

- *Enrolment* is the process in which participants take on different roles and functions in the network. Organizing the network is central to this concept.

- *Mobility* is about the extent to which the participants create a common identity and allow others to represent them and how they speak for the network externally.

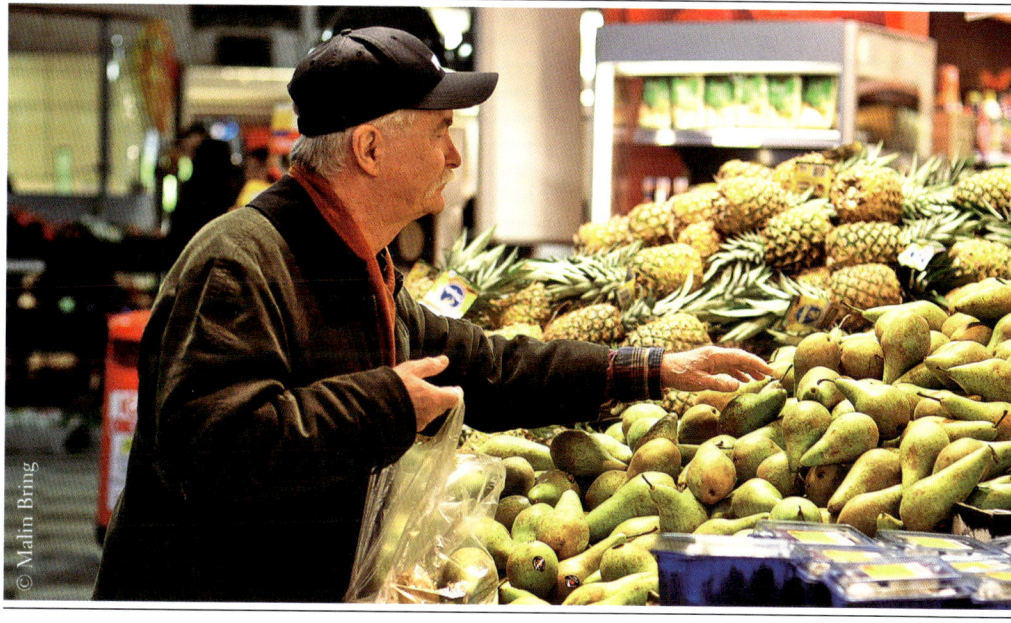

The reasoning around the concept of visualization and the four network forming concepts converges into the conclusion that establishing a strong network around a common visualization will create legitimacy for the visualization.

Section 3. Theoretical framework

Section 4. Addressing health inequities in Västra Götaland

This section accounts for the Commission's work including organizational structure, work phases and the scope of the Action Plan that Region Västra Götaland used in its process to address health inequities. Then, the expected results and the outcome are summarized and discussed. The objective of the Commission was to identify the concrete actions that were the most likely, given current knowledge, to reduce health inequalities in the region.
But first, what motivated the assignment?

Motivation

A number of different aspects when taken together could explain the motivation for this process. In Sweden, there is a national public health goal to create the social conditions needed to ensure good health on equal terms for the entire population. This goal was formulated in 2003 and is defined by eleven subgoals that include societal as well as lifestyle-related characteristics. These goals can be viewed as a first step towards a more welfare-oriented public health work (16).

The final report from the WHO Commission on Social Determinants of Health in 2008 started a discussion in Västra Götaland as it did in many other areas across Europe on health equity and fairness in the distribution of the social determinants (3).

Complementary reports were published that explained the societal costs for health inequities and the media/public became aware of the unexpectedly great differences in life expectancies between city areas for example (2). The increased professional knowledge and interest in gathering and presenting statistics and a better understanding of the causes, together with the political will and public awareness, all acted as inspiration for the Commission.

In parallel to the development within the field of health equity, the concept of social sustainability appeared on the agenda of public authorities as well as in research and media. As inequalities in society became tangible and the effects of people's dissatisfaction spread from one neighbourhood to another, the social aspects of sustainability became more pressing for stakeholders in all domains and spheres – for public authorities as well as nongovernmental organizations.

The regional organization with public health as a field between (1) health and medical care and (2) regional development was a vital arena for including stakeholders in the work that followed. Bridging both pillars of the regional responsibilities is crucial, since the question of social sustainability and health equity relies on both of these arenas.

Organizational structure

The organizational structure of the Commission had two objectives: (1) to anchor its work in the internal organization at the political level as well as at the administrative level and (2) to include a broad spectrum of stakeholders by using a bottom-up approach. The Regional Council decision in 2010 was the precondition for the first objective, where internal stakeholders were named. The Commission was thus led by *a Political Steering Group* represented by politicians from the HMCCs, the Regional Development Committee, the Cultural Affairs Committee and the Human Rights Committee. The Commission was chaired by the Chair of the Public Health Committee. The Steering Group met on a regular basis and gave feedback on the work that was carried out by the other arenas working with the Action Plan, mainly the project group and working group. This was an important part of the internal anchoring to get everyone on board.

For anchoring at administrative level as well as enabling the professional level to be an active part in the organizational structure, a *workgroup or task force* was also formed. The workgroup comprised officials from the aforementioned administrations and representatives for some of the municipalities in Västra Götaland, the Coordination Association, the Swedish Public Employment Service, the Social Insurance Office, the County Administrative Board of Västra Götaland, trade union organizations and the non-profit sector. Parties outside the Region's organization participated on a voluntary basis and according to their own assignments. These representatives were also supposed to report back and anchor in their own organizations as well as provide input on the work.

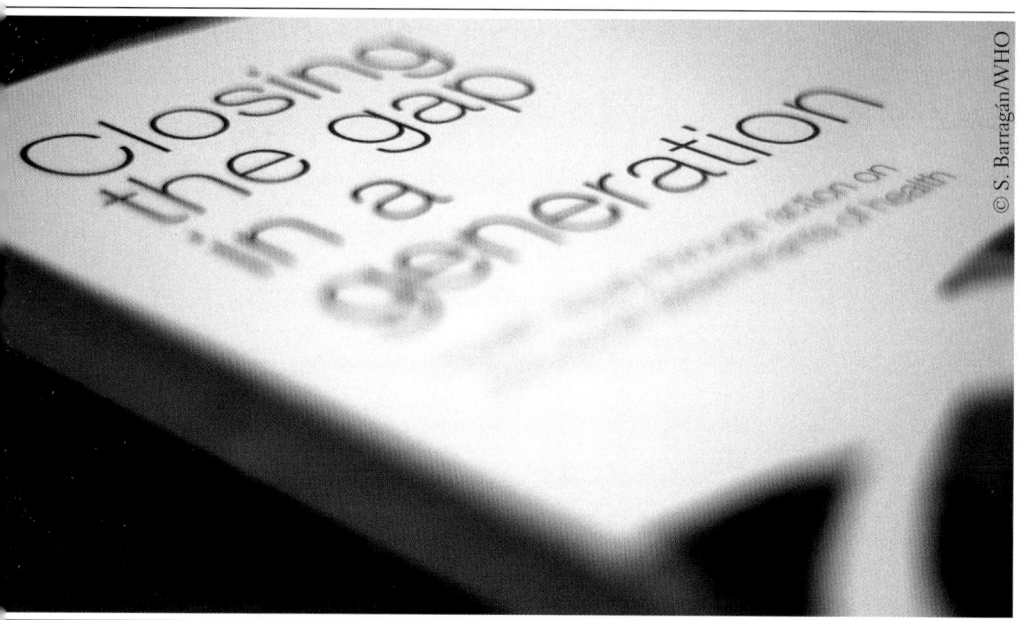

In order to attain a broad and geographical spread, reference groups and reference networks were consulted. Representation from the national level was lacking. Instead the Swedish Association of Local Authorities and Regions through its network "Joint Action for Social Sustainability – Reduce Differences in Health" – where in total 20 regions, county councils and municipalities participated – acted as the national geographical representation. International networks, such as the WHO Regions for Health Network and European Union projects (Joint Action/Equity Action and PROGRESS ReTHI) with links to health equity also served as reference groups (Fig. 2).

Most of the executive work was done at the Public Health Secretariat, where a project group was formed. This group was in charge of contact with all the other stakeholders and was supposed to function as a link between the rest of the Secretariat and all other groups.

PHASES

The formulation of the Action Plan was a five-phase process (Fig. 3). And as with the organizational structure, the purpose was to anchor the work and involve more stakeholders who could participate in preparing as well as implementing measures for reducing health inequity.

Fig.2. Organizational structure of the Commission

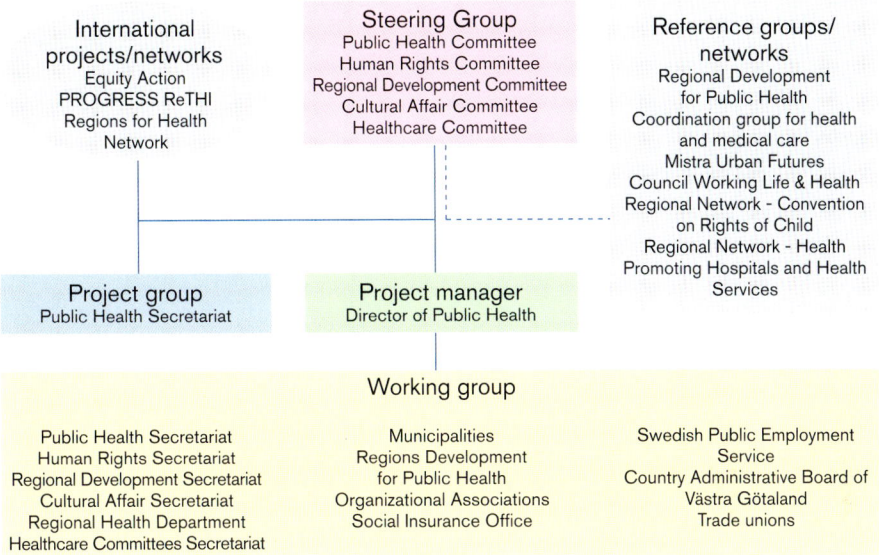

Source: adapted and reproduced by permission from Region Västra Götaland *(4)*.

The Public Health Committee used a bottom-up-approach when it led a previous commission for its regional public health policy *(20)*. Since that approach worked well, it decided to use a similar model – including the same means to anchor and mobilize stakeholders in the work – for the Commission to create the Action Plan, which resulted in the organizational structure in Fig.2.

PLANNING PHASE (2010→)

- The workplan and project organization were outlined by the Public Health Committee, the project manager and the project group.
- An election in Västra Götaland and other events postponed the launch of the project. Since the Commission was put into place before the election, it did not jeopardize the anticipated work but had an impact on the set timeframe.

Section 4. Addressing health inequities in Västra Götaland

Fig.3. Timeline and phases used by the Commission

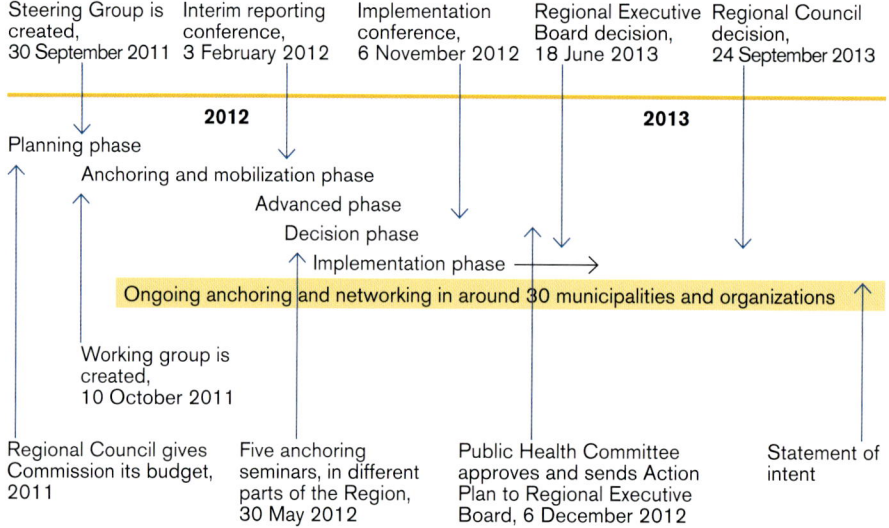

Source: adapted and reproduced by permission from Region Västra Götaland (4).

ANCHORAGE AND MOBILIZATION PHASE (2011→)

- The Steering Group was formed in accordance with the Commission.

- The Steering Group and the project group selected and invited participants in the workgroup.

- The Steering Group's first assignment was to formulate and operationalize the target for the Commission.

- In February 2012, the first interim reporting took place in the form of a conference, where actors from different organizations in Västra Götaland were invited to propose relevant situations and measures to be included in the process.

ADVANCED PHASE (SPRING 2012)

- The project group formulated proposals.
- These were then revised based on discussions in the workgroup.

- Reference networks were consulted.
- Dialogue seminars across Västra Götaland were also held to reach more stakeholders and especially other municipalities than the ones represented in the workgroup.

Decision phase (mid-autumn 2012 – spring 2013)

- A conference was held in Gothenburg for a broad spectrum of stakeholders to view the result of the combined work and have a final say on it.
- The Public Health Committee unanimously approved the Action Plan in early December 2012.
- The Action Plan was sent to the Regional Executive Board for approval during the spring of 2013, and a last official consultation was carried out in the municipalities.
- In early autumn 2013, the Regional Counsel approved the framework, which now applies as a steering document for the entire regional organization.

Implementation phase (autumn 2013→)

- The Public Health Committee and its secretariat will continue having responsibility for coordinating, communicating, measuring and initiating the Action Plan.
- The continued involvement of other stakeholders will be achieved with, among others, the use of declarations of intent.[3]

Action Plan

The Action Plan was to be a document that could act as a concretization of the regional public health policy *(20)* as well as a regional version of the WHO report *Closing the gap in a generation (3)*. The workgroup identified

---

[3] A more detailed description is in Section 4.

situations that were judged to be the most urgent in terms of health inequities. The situations were first agreed upon in the different groups and networks and afterwards complemented with statistical descriptions and a research summary. Then, the situations were organized in accordance with the three challenges in the regional public health policy that have a life-course perspective: *safe and satisfactory early-life conditions, increased participation in working life and ageing with quality of life*. The two challenges that have a more general character – *creating conditions for good living habits* and *lifelong learning* – were integrated into these three challenges (20).

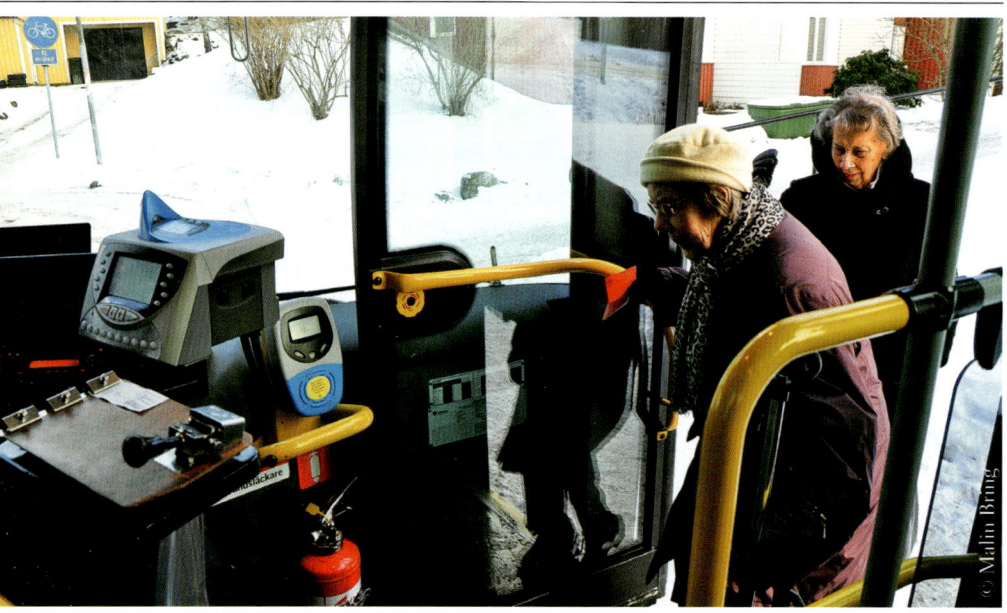

Since the regional public health policy already was a regional steering document and the challenges in implementing it have influenced Västra Götaland's public health work, it was natural to organize the situations and measures that followed around it.

Within each situation, measures that were judged to have the potential to impact the situation in a favourable direction were selected. These represent a selection of the several hundred proposals that have been collected during the work. Early on, a research group was to be formed with the purpose of discussing the validity of the suggested measures. This was not compatible with the idea of a grassroots anchoring, and thus the measures were validated by professionals. Every situation has between 2–5 measures linked to it, and a number of different stakeholders are indirectly incorporated into the future work as a result of the nature of the suggested measures.

In addition to the measures along the life-course perspective, a sustainable formal structure is necessary to coordinate actions among the different responsible authorities. Knowledge development in the areas of social sustainability and health equity and systems monitoring health equity in Västra Götaland are also of particular importance and are included in the Action Plan *(4)*.

During a discussion that took place at the Regional Council meeting (January 2013), certain paragraphs in the Action Plan were scrutinized and criticized by the political opposition; the arguments being the lack of accountability an individual has for his or her own health as compared to the strong emphasis on structural, upstream health determinants. The opposition called for a better balance between structural and individual approaches. Members in the majority ran into difficulties handling this criticism. They wanted a unanimous decision in support of the Action Plan to pass it to the Regional Council in order for the Action Plan to be sustainable over several mandate periods. This disagreement launched a period of negotiations and also included a request for comments from the 49 municipalities within the Region to ensure that they were supportive. This period lasted 6 months but strengthened the Action Plan since the support from the municipalities was documented. In September 2013, the Action Plan was unanimously approved by the Regional Council.

Implementation through declarations of intent

The result of the Commission is a framework that intends to be a tool and guide for work towards health equity. Each actor takes decisions into his or her own organization on which of the proposed initiatives/measures should be implemented, together with whom, when and how. To focus the combined efforts, a tool called declarations of intent will be used. These will act as agreements between the various actors who want to commit themselves to work in accordance with the Action Plan. Depending on the combination of partners, each declaration will vary in degree of concreteness.

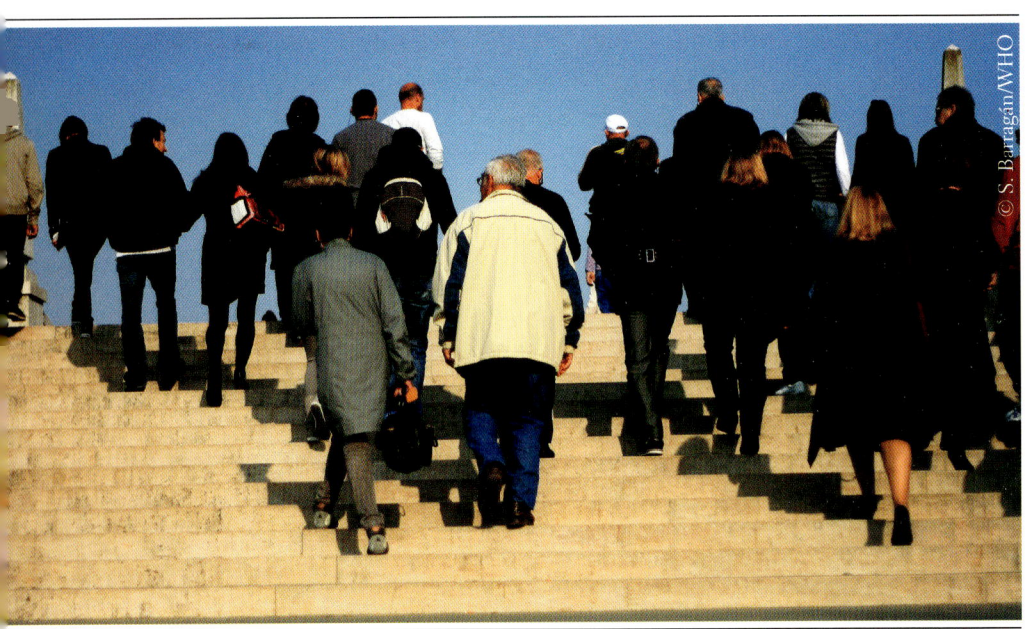

The common denominator in all of these declarations is that they should contain actions that aim towards health equity. Each declaration of intent will consist of a more general section, where the guiding principles and a common framework will be given. This will be followed by a more specified section listing concrete actions on which the agreement will focus. An important aspect of future work is how to follow up and evaluate implementation, which will also be included in the declaration. Lastly, a general idea for next steps and future handling of the results will also be included.

INFLUENCES ON THE COMMISSION AND ITS OUTCOME

This subsection focuses on a number of factors affecting the Commission as well as the outcome, with the help of the theoretical framework.

TIMING

As Kingdon states, there is a window of opportunity for policy-making, by using the three streams: problem, policy and political *(17)*. With the WHO report on creating health equity by focusing on the social determinants of problem with health inequalities became more visible (3). Regional reports stating the costs and existence of health inequalities as well as initiatives within the Region provided even more insight (2). As the problem of increasing gaps in society grew clearer and the public awareness stronger, there was political will to act. Lastly, as can be seen below, different departments (that would become connected to the work within the Commission) were already prepared to work towards a comprehensive policy.

In the WHO report (8), five reasons for working with health equity are listed, varying from the individual rights perspective to economic incentives. As a complementary explanation to the question of "Why now?", the regional organizations had clearly taken steps to recognize the reasons. For example, the creation of a Human Rights Committee had put focus on the human rights issue; the social risks were becoming more present and were already accepted by national authorities as well as regional bodies as valid risks; and, finally, the connection between health equity and societal resources and sustainability had been established.

Understanding the results

The work of the Commission has a clear connection to what Callon calls network formation (19, 21). By using the four "moments of translation", some major decisions as well as outcomes become more visible and easy to understand.

Problematization focuses on the question of who was included in the network, which in turn is a result of how the purpose and scope are presented and communicated. Public health work in Västra Götaland has a long history of intersectional organizations, with public as well as civic organizations. The Steering Group consisted of regional politicians who were commissioned to participate. The level of knowledge and interest in the area of social sustainability and health equity varied, which can be seen both in the attendance records as well as the political discussions that arose during the decision phase. The workgroup was principally a network of stakeholders who attended on a voluntary basis. Most of the representatives already had an interest in public health and could easily recognize the problematizations. However, the concept of health inequalities proved to be an obstacle to full commitment to the joint venture since several of the stakeholders were not explicitly dealing with health issues as part of their missions. For example, the statutes of the Public Employment Service do not contain health issues explicitly even if unemployment is at the core as a social determinant for health, which is also biased towards those at the lower end of the social ladder. On the other hand, the concept of social sustainability proved to be the key to an agreement on joint action against the unfair distribution of the social determinants of health.

Interessement can be closely linked to the problematization process. A major advantage in terms of the workgroup was that many of the representatives already were involved or enrolled in similar work. Participating in the Commission was a way to boost the public health work and provide concrete measures to include in their own work. The process also ensured participation where all stakeholders could provide/suggest situations and measures. One practical problem occurred when the many suggestions had to be reduced. A way to handle this particular problem was the term "live document", which meant that this framework consisted of some relevant measures but that it could be revised as knowledge within this area developed.

In terms of the Steering Group, the situation was different, since it was not only one's own interest or previous engagement that was the reason for involvement. As work progressed, the Steering Group developed the idea of creating some common ground so the mandate for the Action Plan would not change even if the political landscape did. It was, thus, very important to try incorporating different political interests. An example is the distinction and connection between the individuals with responsibility for their health versus societal responsibility for the health of the population. Describing situations was not as politically challenging as suggesting concrete ways to change them. The idea of the Action Plan as a portfolio instead of a checklist developed as a way to handle this. The suggested measures could be seen as one way to affect health equity in a favourable direction but not the only way.

During the process, the intention was to involve a research group and a broader network of municipalities. The purpose of the research network was to validate the suggested measures and to provide input on prioritizing them. At an initial meeting, the research network was sceptical to the suggested purpose and the nature of the measures and was also concerned that the researchers could be used as alibis to justify suggestions that they did not approve. Obviously there was, to some extent, a lack of trust in the Commission, implying that the Commission was not successful in its dialogue at that time.

Another difficulty was to find appropriate representation from the 49 municipalities in the Region. Their socioeconomic context differs, as does their capacity to organize efficient welfare strategies, since the variation in their economic structure differs.

Overall, the way to create interest in the areas of social sustainability and health equity was by using incentives rather than coercion, especially since there was no overarching authority that could decide for all stakeholders. Instead what prevailed in *interessement* was the idea that the Action Plan would be of use for all stakeholders in some way.

Enrolment and mobilization focus on the different functions among the stakeholders and the mechanisms that seem important for strengthening the network. Besides the project group who carried the executive role and acted as an engine in this process, there are three arenas that are important. Firstly, the Steering Group functioned as an overarching assembly where strategic crossroads were handled. It also played an important role for the political anchoring that later paved the way for approval by the Regional Council, even though the political road offered more obstacles than expected. A second arena was the workgroup who during the process had two major functions: (1) to provide suggestions and, later on, to anchor the preliminary plan; and (2) to play a significant role as spokespersons for implementation. The workgroup became the hub of the network. The third arena was the conferences and dialogue seminars that, in a general way, had the same functions as the workgroup.

Generally the Commission managed to enrol and mobilize engaged stakeholders, but there were some politicians as well as officials that did not anchor the work in the network in their own organizations. One reason for this could be inadequate mandates from their organizations, as well as lack of interest. Another reason might be that the enrolment in this joint process is but one of the tasks that occupy the representatives in the workgroup.

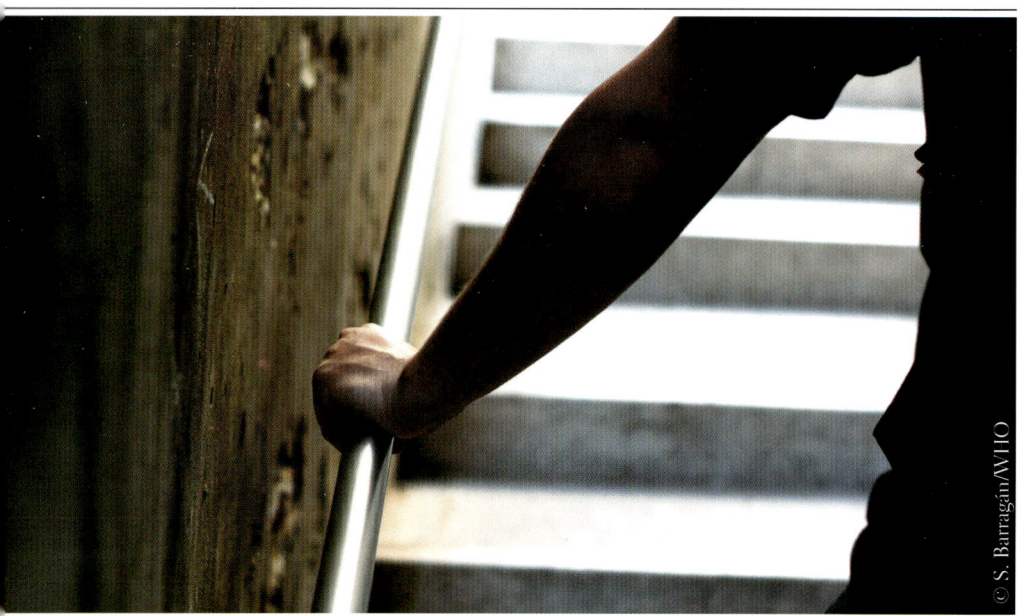

Future work

For future work and a successful implementation, there are some conditions that will play a significant role. Positive factors include the establishment of a politically approved Action Plan and a broad network of stakeholders that all have assignments within the field of social sustainability and health equity.

Of more interest might be the conditions that could be challenging for future success. Firstly, there is a major difference in the level of political interest among stakeholders. Secondly, there are ideological differences in relation to the idea of what needs and can be done. This is most visible in discussions around actions that require financial priorities, especially when it comes to the balance between distal and proximate actions, the individual's own responsibility for his or her health. Thirdly, a gap exists between the policy level and the stakeholders closer to the service level, which means that there is no clear decision and/or delivery chain *(8)*. Lastly, a policy document can be viewed in different ways and so can this Action Plan. The Action Plan is supposed to be a tool to facilitate cooperation between stakeholders, and to be evaluated and supplemented as knowledge about this area develops and new measures are proposed. This requires means to evaluate and measure effects but also a fair amount of flexibility and resources to be able to keep this Action Plan in line with other prioritized political issues that are on the agenda or in other existing policy documents. These other prioritized issues could be health care, education, and support to major research initiatives or creating good environments for smaller businesses.

Section 5. Discussion

When engaging in smart governance processes that extend over different public sectors as well as the political sphere and civic society, a lot of time and energy will have to focus on finding tools for cooperation and mutual understanding. As a summary, some of the possibilities and difficulties encountered are discussed.

The concept of health inequalities proved to be a difficult concept to form a network of different stakeholders around. Instead social sustainability became the common denominator among stakeholders. A number of the workgroup members thought it might be difficult to establish their contribution to the network if health inequalities should be the core concept, since the statutes of their organizations did not explicitly deal with health. However, no one found a similar difficulty with social sustainability. Given that growing health inequalities are incompatible with socially sustainable development, the Commission agreed that the core concept of the process should be collaboration for social sustainability. This is an example of the importance of a common terminology. Finding and agreeing to this language are critical means through which the participants communicate their expectations on the upcoming process and the preconditions for them to legitimize their participation. This proved to be useful also to link actions against health inequalities to regional development policies, which often use the rhetoric around sustainable development as a foundation, thereby enabling a communicative channel to other actors not yet involved in the process.

One main conclusion from reviews and strategies to tackle health inequalities is that politicians need to be involved and to be advocates of actions; if health inequalities are not on the political agenda, no political decisions will be made to reduce them and, consequently, no action will be taken. But soon enough this endeavour will be challenged. The counterarguments are rarely about the intention to reduce unfair health disparities but rather about the means to get there. This is illustrated in the process when the Action Plan was to be approved within the Regional Executive Board and passed to the Regional Council. Even if the political disagreement was unexpected – the Steering Group had representatives of both the majority and the opposition – and caused a delay, the final decision in the Regional Council would probably not have been possible without the commitment of the Steering Group.

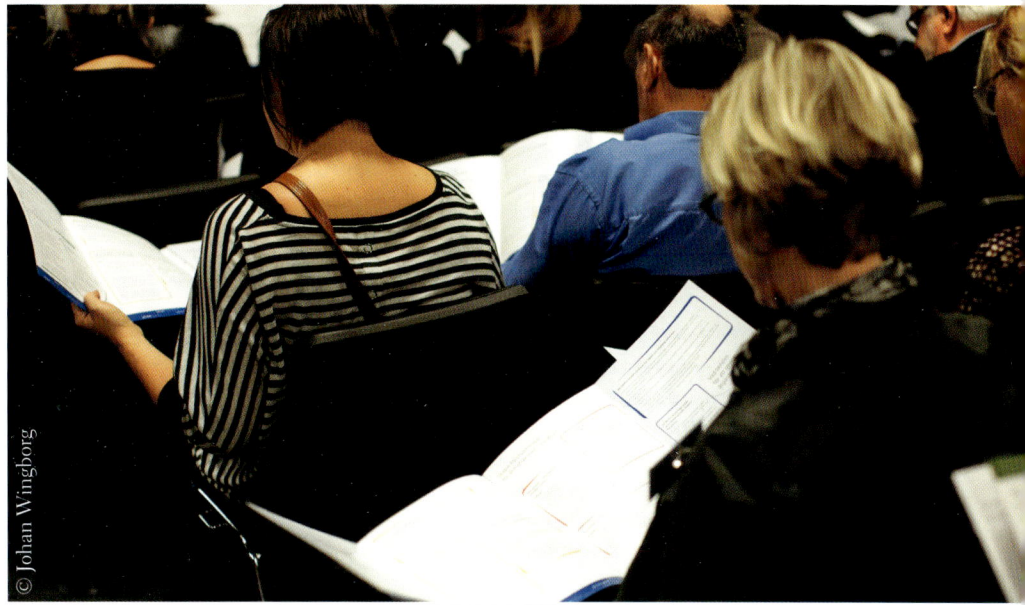

The process in Västra Götaland proved in a way to be a compromise: on the one hand, it was judged as necessary to gather participants from politics, practice and theory (research) around the same table to develop an action plan; on the other hand, it proved not to be possible to enrol the research community fully into the process. According to the evaluation, this was the result from the pressure to keep to the time schedule; it was simply too complex an endeavour to integrate the three perspectives within the given timeframe. Meeting the schedule was prioritized above including researchers in order to meet expectations at political level and from the workgroup. Instead, the establishment of a platform where researchers, politicians and practitioners could meet was identified as a strategic objective to be prioritized and achieved as part of the Action Plan, according to the Regional Council decision.

A stronger link to the research community would probably have allowed scientists to present evidenced-based research and practices in Västra Götaland and might have shortened the six-month delay in approving the Action Plan. Instead, information from other reviews, for example the Commission for a Socially Sustainable Malmö (6) and the WHO Commission on Social Determinants of Health (3), was collected and translated into a regional context for Västra Götaland and presented to the politicians by the secretariats and workgroup, who did not have the same authority as the scientists.

Another aspect of the lack of scientific backup during the process is that the proposed actions were based on the knowledge and experiences within the workgroup and other contributors. These actions tended to be identified with the perspective of the different stakeholders and based on their objectives and agendas. This might lead to a near-sighted set of suggestions, which might run the risk of being too close to the individual, and thus not have sufficient impact on the causes of the causes, i.e. the structures and mechanisms that create health inequalities. On the other hand, an overemphasis on scientific evidence-based information for the suggested actions might run the risk of being too abstract and leaving the practitioners and politicians without a proper understanding of how such actions should be implemented. Ideally, the actions should be scientifically sound, and discussed and negotiated among scientists, politicians and practitioners, so it is crucial to find out how such a dialogue could be realized.

One final aspect of this triangulation between practitioners, politicians and researchers can be linked to Knaggård's (22) argumentation when studying Swedish policy-making relating to climate issue and scientific uncertainty. A certain level of scientific uncertainty can provide a common platform for cooperation due to the fact that the uncertainty provides room for interpretation and the possibility to adapt the new challenge into already existing policies. This might have been the case with the concept of *social sustainability* and the lack of a coherent researcher community connected to the process.

A checklist to complete before starting the process of creating an action plan to address health inequities includes answering certain questions.

- Is there a political mandate and/or political support?
- Are all relevant stakeholders included in the process? If it is not possible, are there ways to inform and/or include them or their comments in the future?
- Does everyone know his or her expected role in the process? Is this role anchored in one's home organization?
- Has a commonly agreed goal been set?
- Is the goal as concrete as possible?

- Has a method for the process been agreed upon and does it suit the aim?
- Is terminology agreed upon and/or is the problem/challenge described in a way that includes and engages all stakeholders?
- Have discussions taken place and/or has a plan been made for future challenges such as delivery chains, decision fora and future responsibilities?
- How will the policy/action plan be evaluated – as a whole and/or piecemeal?
- Before finalization, how does this action plan connect/relate to other steering documents?

References[4]

1. Danielsson M, Talbäck M. Public health: an overview: health in Sweden: The National Public Health Report 2012. Chapter 1. Scand J Public Health. 2012;40:6–22. doi: 10.1177/1403494812459457.

2. Calidoni F, Christiansson C, Henriksson G. Kostnader för ojämlikhet i hälsa i Västra Götaland [Costs of health inequalities in Västra Götaland]. Göteborg: Region Västra Götaland; 2011 (in Swedish) (http://www.vgregion.se/upload/Folkh%c3%a4lsa/j%c3%a4mlik%20h%c3%a4lsa/SlutrapportOj%c3%a4mlikhetskostnadeVGR.pdf).

3. Commission on Social Determinants of Health. Closing the gap in a generation: health equity through action on the social determinants of health. Final Report of the Commission on Social Determinants of Health. Geneva: World Health Organization; 2008 (http://www.who.int/social_determinants/thecommission/finalreport/en/).

4. Together towards Social Sustainability. Action Plan for Health Equity in Region Västra Götaland, Sweden. Göteborg: Region Västra Götaland; 2013 (http://www.aer.eu/fileadmin/user_upload/Programmes/Breakfast_briefings/BB_13_05_15/Handlingsplan_eng_130215.pdf).

5. Strand M, Brown C, Torgersen TP, Giæver Ø. Setting the political agenda to tackle health inequity in Norway. Copenhagen: WHO Regional Office for Europe; 2009 (Studies on social and economic determinants of population health, No 4; http://www.euro.who.int/__data/assets/pdf_file/0014/110228/E93431.pdf).

6. Stigendal M, Östergren P-O, editors. Malmö's path towards a sustainable future, third edition. Malmö: Commission for a Socially Sustainable Malmö; 2013 (http://www.malmo.se/download/18.51821d07143bab87ba7c4ac/1392805314379/malm%C3%B6kommisionen_rapport_engelsk_web.pdf).

7. Health 2020. A European policy framework and strategy for the 21st century. Copenhagen: WHO Regional Office for Europe; 2013 (http://www.euro.who.int/en/health-topics/health-policy/health-2020-the-european-policy-for-health-and-well-being/publications/2013/health-2020-a-european-policy-framework-and-strategy-for-the-21st-century).

8. Brown C, Harrison D, Burns H, Ziglio E. Governance for health equity. Taking forward the equity values and goals of Health 2020 in the WHO European Region. Copenhagen: WHO Regional Office for Europe: 2014 (http://www.euro.who.int/__data/assets/pdf_file/0020/235712/e96954.pdf).

---

4 All websites accessed on 12 June 2014.

9. About Region Västra Götaland. In Region Västra Götaland [website] Göteborg: Region Västra Götaland; 2013 (http://www.vgregion.se/en/Vastra-Gotalandsregionen/Home/About-us/).

10. Förslag till detaljutformning av den politiska organisationen 2015–2018. Diarienummer RS 691-2012 [Proposal for a detailed design of the political organization 2015–2018]. Göteborg: Region Västra Götaland; 2014 (in Swedish).

11. Protokoll från regionfullmäktige, 2014-04-15. [Protocol from Regional Council, 2014-04-15]. Göteborg: Region Västra Götaland; 2014 (in Swedish).

12. Kickbusch I, Gleicher D. Governance for health in the 21st century. Copenhagen: WHO Regional Office for Europe; 2012 (http://www.euro.who.int/__data/assets/pdf_file/0019/171334/RC62BD01-Governance-for-Health-Web.pdf).

13. Bambra C, Joyce KE, Bellis MA, Greatley A, Greengross S, Hughes S, et al. Reducing health inequalities in priority public health conditions: using rapid review to develop proposals for evidence-based policy. J Public Health (Oxf). 2010; 32(4):496–505. doi: 10.1093/pubmed/fdq028.

14. Bengtsson M. Att genomföra politiska beslut: varför blir det som det blir när vi vill så väl. Forskningsöversikt och diskussionsunderlag, november 2012 [Implementing policy decisions: why is it that things are the way they are when our intentions are good. Research and Discussion Paper, November 2012]. Research overview for Knowledge about and Approaches to Fair and Socially Sustainable Cities (KAIROS), Mistra Urban Futures. Göteborg: School of Public Administration, Göteborg University; 2012 (in Swedish) (http://www.mistraurbanfutures.org/sites/default/files/visioner_och_deras_genomforande_0.pdf).

15. Kouzes JM, Mico PR. Domain Theory: An Introduction to Organizational Behavior in Human Service Organizations. J Appl Behav Sci. 1979; 15:449–469. doi: 10.1177/002188637901500402.

16. Ten years of Swedish public health policy – Summary report. Swedish National Institute of Public Health. Östersund: Swedish National Institute of Public Health; 2013.

17. Kingdon JW. Agendas, alternatives, and public policies. Boston: Longman; 2011.

18. Latour B. Visualisation and cognition: thinking with eyes and hands. In: Kucklick H, editor. Knowledge and society studies in the sociology of culture past and present. Greenwood: Jai Press; 1986: 1–40.

19. Callon M. Some elements of a sociology of translation: domestication of the scallops and the fishermen of St Brieuc Bay. In: Law J, editor. Power, action and belief: a new sociology of knowledge?. London: Routledge; 1986: 196–223.

20. Public health policy Västra Götaland. Mariestad: Region Västra Götaland; 2009 (http://www.vgregion.se/upload/Folkh%c3%a4lsa/policy/Folkh%c3%a4lsopolitisk%20policy%20engelsk_Tillg%c3%a4nglig.pdf).

21. Kastberg G. Organisering i nätverk – en studie av de organisatoriska processerna kring framtagandet av en handlingsplan för en mer jämlik folkhälsa [Organizing in networks – a study of organizational processes related to the development of an action plan for a more equitable public health]. Göteborg: Kommunforskning i Västsverige; 2013 (in Swedish).

22. Knaggård Å. What do policy-makers do with scientific uncertainty? The incremental character of Swedish climate change policy-making. Policy Studies. 2013; 35(1):22–39;. doi:10.1080/01442872.2013.804175 (http://www.tandfonline.com/doi/abs/10.1080/01442872.2013.804175#.U5omovldX74?).